The Drug Abuse Prevention Library

Antidepressants

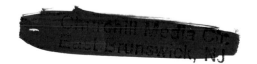

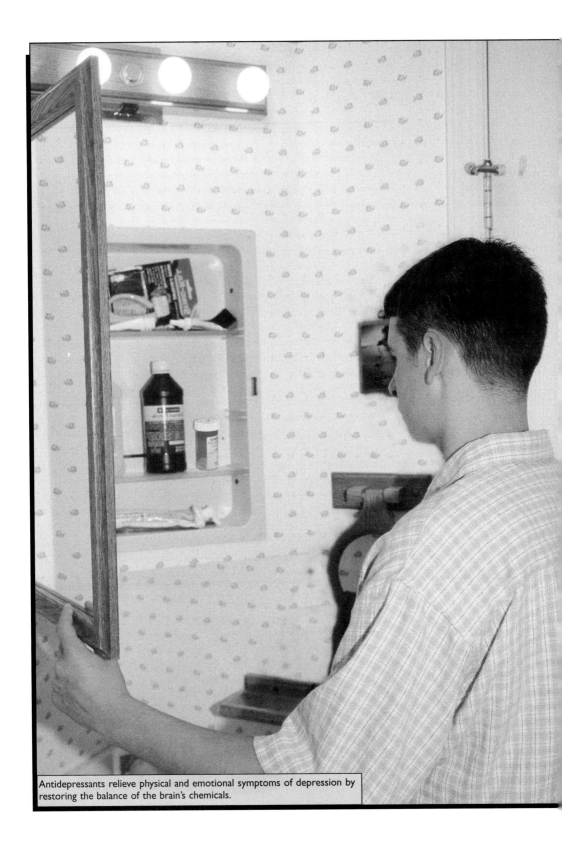

Antidepressants relieve physical and emotional symptoms of depression by restoring the balance of the brain's chemicals.

The Drug Abuse Prevention Library

Antidepressants

Holly Cefrey

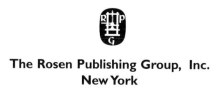

The Rosen Publishing Group, Inc.
New York

To Richard, Elaine, Ethan, and Dean.

Special thanks to the inspirational Rosen group.

The people pictured in this book are only models. They in no way practice or endorse the activities illustrated. Captions serve only to explain the subjects of photographs and do not in any way imply a connection between the real-life models and the staged situations.

Published in 2000 by The Rosen Publishing Group, Inc.
29 East 21st Street, New York, NY 10010

Cefrey, Holly.
    Antidepressants: / Holly Cefrey.
        p. cm. — (The drug abuse prevention library)
    Includes bibliographical references and index.
    ISBN 0-8239-3283-4 (lib. bdg.)
        1. Antidepressants—Juvenile literature.
    [1. Antidepressants.] I. Title. II. Series.
    2000
    362.2—dc21

Manufactured in the United States of America

Contents

Introduction

"*The simple fact is that I had changed. Looking back, it's easy to see why we missed the signs that I was severely depressed. My parents thought that it was a phase. While our bodies are changing, teens experience a lot of different emotions, but mine were mostly sadness, hopelessness, and anger. I was so depressed that eventually I would need medication to help me find my way back to an easier life.*

"*My parents started to call me mood man. The truth is that I really was moody. Everything was upsetting to me. I was irritable for no obvious reason and it did not let up. I even started acting out at school. Before my depression I loved playing sports. During my depression I would often skip practice. When I did make it I found myself snapping at the coach and my teammates. I did not know how to tell anyone about what was going on inside of me.*

"I started to feel really tired and I had terrible headaches. They were so bad that I thought of killing myself. I wasn't as close to my friends as I used to be and when I told them that life was not worth living, I frightened them even more. Luckily one of my friends told my dad. My parents took me to a psychiatrist who treats only children and teens. This type of doctor is specially trained to understand and treat the problems that we go through. My doctor diagnosed me with major depression and prescribed a medication to help me."

—Nathan, seventeen

Nathan was suffering from depression. Depression is a real and serious illness that anyone can develop—even children and teens. Several well-known figures have suffered from depression, ranging from Abraham Lincoln and Winston Churchill to Vincent Van Gogh. Depression is much more than feeling low or sad. It actually changes the balance of chemicals in the brain. When the chemicals of the brain are out of balance, it can affect the brain's thought processes as well as the rest of the

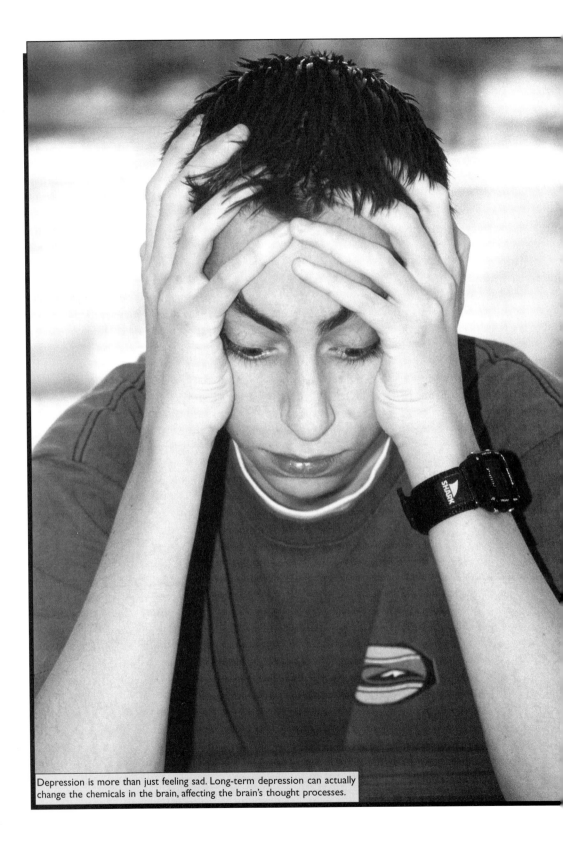

Depression is more than just feeling sad. Long-term depression can actually change the chemicals in the brain, affecting the brain's thought processes.

body. Depression can change how you normally act. It can also alter the way you feel about yourself, other people, and everything else in your life. It can affect eating, sleeping, and studying habits.

There are different kinds of depression. Each depression affects people differently. The symptoms (signs of an illness) of depression are different in each person. Some depressions are mild, while others are very serious and long lasting. The treatment plan, or therapy, that a psychologist or psychiatrist may choose varies for each patient. Psychologists treat their patients with a variety of psychotherapies (therapy by talking). Psychiatrists are doctors of medicine and are trained in the use of medication to treat depression. The kind of depression that you have, and the severity of how it affects your life, will determine what type of treatment you will receive.

Many people who have depression don't even know that they have it. They may believe that depression occurs only when something bad or sad has happened, but depression can develop without any triggers. Untreated, depression can cause other serious health problems. Some depressions left untreated can lead to suicide, which is why treatment of even mild depression is very important. Above all, it is important to remember that suffering from depression is not a sign of weakness, and when treated, it will hopefully get better.

The treatment for Nathan's depression was a medication known as an antidepressant. Antidepressants work to relieve the physical and emotional symptoms of depression. It is believed that antidepressants work by bringing back the balance of chemicals in the brain. This book will explain the use and effects of antidepressants in the treatment of depression. For further exploration of depression and antidepressants, you can refer to the Where to Go for Help and For Further Reading sections of this book.

Understanding Antidepressants

The battle that a person wages against depression begins long before it is actually treated. As stated in the introduction, people with depression can be suffering without knowing it. It is even more difficult to diagnose depression in children and adolescents. Studies have shown that the symptoms of a depressive disorder (such as Nathan's) are often mistaken for normal mood swings that are typical during childhood and adolescent development. Children and teens also find it difficult to discuss what is happening. Many youths tell themselves that the way they feel must be normal, otherwise someone would be helping them. If you are at the stage where you are getting treated for depression—that is an accomplishment in itself—your battle is half over.

Clarifying the Controversy About Antidepressant Medication

When the medical profession prescribes a medication as a treatment, the medication has already been put through a number of tests and research studies to prove that it is safe and effective. Safe medication means that it will not cause harm to the patient, and effective medication means that it works well without adding too many unwanted side effects. The research findings for antidepressant medication show that it is a safe and effective treatment for depression in adults. Using antidepressants to treat children and teens, however, has been the cause of some controversy in the medical profession.

This controversy revolves around the fact that antidepressants are being prescribed for youths without a great deal of research to support the long-term effectiveness of antidepressants for treatment of adolescent depression. The lack of research is due to the fact that prescribing antidepressants to treat children and teens is a relatively new therapy. Some short-term studies, however, have shown that antidepressants are safe and effective

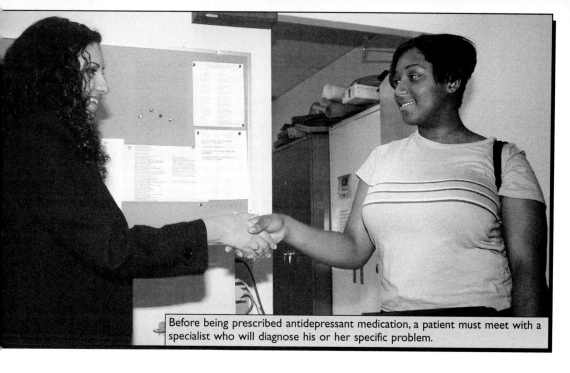

Before being prescribed antidepressant medication, a patient must meet with a specialist who will diagnose his or her specific problem.

for use by children and teens with depression. Large-scale, long-term research is still needed, though, to show which antidepressants work best for youths.

To ensure that a child or teen is given the most currently recommended and researched treatment, it is usually suggested that the youth be evaluated and diagnosed by a psychiatrist or psychologist who specializes in treating children and teens. While it is true that pediatricians and family doctors can prescribe antidepressants, these health professionals are not fully trained to treat mental illnesses such as depression.

How Antidepressants Work

Antidepressants help to balance chemicals in the brain while a person is suffering from depression. The use of antidepressants can lift the dark, isolating moods of depression. They also provide relief for physical symptoms of depression, such as headaches and drained energy levels. By relieving the symptoms of depression, antidepressants can make other kinds of treatment more effective. Some people suffer from a depression so severe that they cannot speak. Antidepressants can allow those people to communicate and to respond to counseling or psychotherapy. Antidepressants can give very depressed people the mental clarity they need in order to work toward getting better.

Antidepressants are used mostly to treat serious depression, but they can also be used for mild depression. Although they may lift the dark moods of depression, antidepressants are not to be confused with stimulants. Stimulants, or amphetamines, are used to increase mental alertness and physical activity. When you use stimulants, you can feel their effect very soon after taking them. It can take days or even weeks before you can feel the effects of antidepressants.

2

Types of Antidepressants

Antidepressants were introduced as a treatment for depression over forty years ago. Today there are around twenty approved antidepressants. Antidepressants are arranged in groups according to what they are made of and how they are thought to work. The antidepressant groups are:

- MAOIs (Monoamine Oxidase Inhibitors)

- TCAs (Tricyclic Antidepressants)

- SSRIs (Selective Serotonin Reuptake Inhibitors)

- Others —

Some doctors or psychiatrists may also label the antidepressants as old or new.

The old antidepressants are the MAOIs and the TCAs. The new ones are SSRIs and Others, which have been discovered within the last ten to fifteen years. The four sections of this chapter list the most commonly prescribed antidepressants of each group along with a description of the group. Please consult chapter 4 to learn about the possible side effects associated with each group and with antidepressants in general.

MAOIs	
Drug Name	**Brand Name**
Phenelzine	Nardil
Tranylcypromine	Parnate
Isocarboxazid	Marplan (recently taken off the market)

MAOIs were the first antidepressants. Their effectiveness at lifting the depressed mood was discovered accidentally. The very first MAOI was discovered during the research and treatment of tuberculosis, or TB. Patients who were given these drugs, although still suffering with TB, experienced elevated moods. Doctors realized that they could use the medication to treat the symptoms of depression rather than TB.

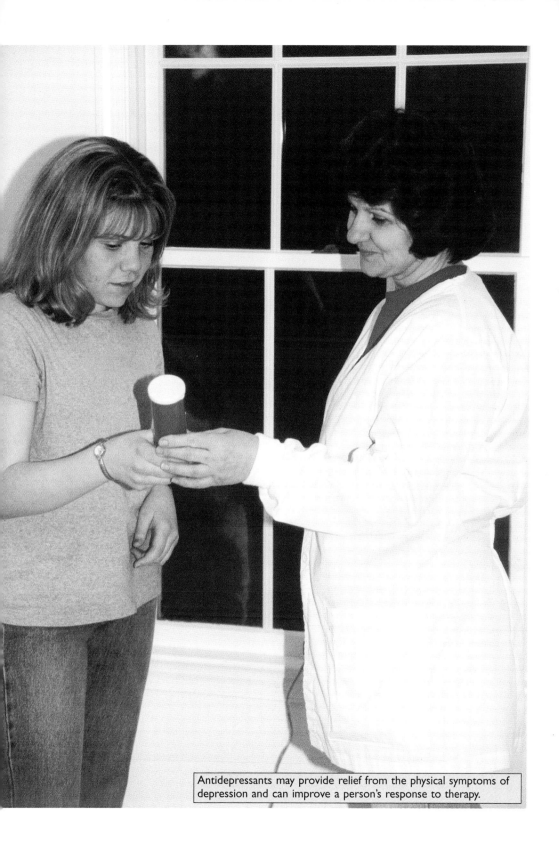

Antidepressants may provide relief from the physical symptoms of depression and can improve a person's response to therapy.

The popularity of prescribing MAOIs for depression has declined in recent years. The decline is due to the side effects brought about by MAOI use, as well as the food and medication restrictions that must be followed while taking these drugs. In some cases, however, MAOIs are still prescribed because they can be extremely effective despite their side effects and restrictions. In fact, many patients who may not get better using the newer antidepressants can be treated successfully with MAOIs. MAOIs are used to treat other mental disorders such as eating disorders and panic or stress disorders.

TCAs	
Drug Name	**Brand Name**
Amitriptyline	Elavil, Endep
Desipramine	Norpramin
Nortriptyline	Pamelor, Aventyl
Trimipramine	Surmontil
Imipramine	Tofranil, Janimine
Protriptyline	Vivactil

TCAs are the second oldest group of antidepressants. TCAs, much like the MAOIs, are used to effectively treat patients who don't get better after using the newer antidepressants. Many psychiatrists prefer to prescribe TCAs instead of MAOIs for patients with major depression because the side effects are often fewer with TCAs. One brand of TCA was the first approved drug to treat obsessive-compulsive disorder, which is now commonly treated with Prozac or Luvox (both are SSRIs). Obsessive-compulsive disorder, or OCD, is a type of anxiety disorder where a person thinks the same thoughts or does the same action repeatedly over a long period of time. Like OCD, a number of other mental disorders can be treated with TCAs.

SSRIs	
Drug Name	**Brand Name**
Fluoxetine	Prozac
Paroxetine	Paxil
Sertraline	Zoloft
Fluvoxamine	Luvox
Citalopram	Celexa

SSRIs are a newer group of antidepressants. They have fewer side effects than the old antidepressants. Because the older antidepressants have such serious side effects, many cases of mild depression were not medically treated. With the discovery of SSRIs, however, doctors have been able to treat even mild depression with antidepressants.

SSRIs are the most commonly prescribed drugs to treat mild to moderate depression in children and teens. Prozac was the very first SSRI, and it was approved for treatment in 1987. In addition to treating depression, SSRIs are used to treat a variety of disorders including anxiety and panic disorders and bulimia. Luvox is approved by the Food and Drug Administration for the use in treatment of obsessive-compulsive disorders (OCDs).

Others	
Drug Name	**Brand Name**
Bupropion	Wellbutrin
Trazodone	Desyrel
Venlafaxine	Effexor
Nefazodone	Serzone
Mirtazapine	Remeron

The newest antidepressants are grouped under the category of Others because they do not fit into the MAOIs,

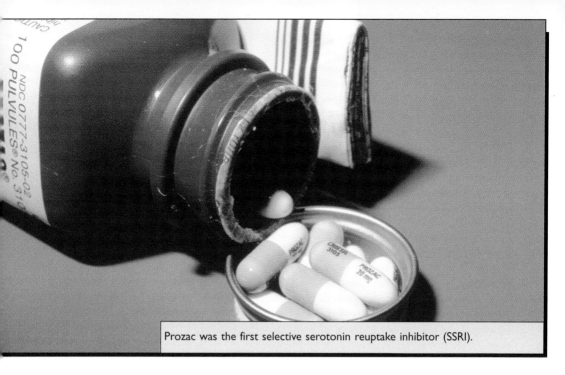

Prozac was the first selective serotonin reuptake inhibitor (SSRI).

TCAs, or SSRIs. They do not fit into the three groups because they are chemically different. Antidepressants of this group seem to have the fewest side effects.

In addition to the four groups of antidepressants previously listed, drugs of other types can be used to treat mental disorders. For example, lithium, which is not an antidepressant but an antimanic, is sometimes prescribed to treat certain kinds of depression.

3

Taking Antidepressants

"The thought that I could take something to help relieve my depression made me feel so hopeful . . . for the first time in a long while. But as I learned the hard way, waiting for the antidepressants to start working can be a confusing and frustrating experience."

—Amy, eighteen

Amy started taking an antidepressant for a two-year-long depression. Almost two weeks had gone by, and even though she was sleeping better, she was still depressed. The possibility that the antidepressants weren't working made Amy feel even more depressed. Her mother had been treated for depression and she had to try two different kinds of antidepressants before the treatment worked. Amy didn't want to go through that; she wanted it to work on the first try.

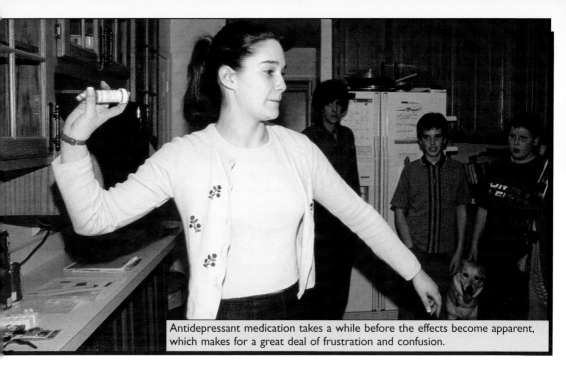

Antidepressant medication takes a while before the effects become apparent, which makes for a great deal of frustration and confusion.

Amy's family kept saying how much better she seemed. It made her feel so much pressure because she didn't feel any different. She started to think that her family was making it all up. She felt as if there was nowhere to turn. At one point, she became so frustrated that she threw her pills at the wall.

"Wow, I can't believe how badly I felt then," she says. "It's a memory that will stay with me forever. In addition to being depressed, I was so frustrated and confused. I thought that the pills might change who I was meant to be. I thought that I would get hooked on them and turn into an antidepressant junkie . . . popping them forever and high all the time. I was scared that if I stopped taking them after I got better, I would return to my murky self.

"What I really needed to do was tell my psychiatrist everything that I was feeling . . . she couldn't read my mind. If she had known all of my fears, she would have helped me to work through them. Talking about your fears can make you feel a lot better about your problems. You might even learn that there isn't anything to worry about."

Amy's fears about antidepressants are not uncommon. Your psychiatrist or doctor will tell you the necessary information about your specific antidepressant, but it's good to ask questions and talk about any concerns that you might have along the way—no matter how unimportant you think they are. When taking a medication, every question or concern is important. Knowing all of the specifics about your medication will allow you to take better care of yourself during your recovery. If for any reason you have been made to feel that you cannot speak freely or ask questions, it's time to get a new psychiatrist or doctor.

Questions and Answers

Although each antidepressant will affect each person differently, here are some general answers to questions about antidepressants. These answers have been proven correct through years of research and study. In addition to these general answers, you can ask your psychiatrist or doctor specific questions about your medication.

Antidepressant questions at a glance

- Are they addictive?

- Will they make me high?

- Will they change who I am?

- How are they given?

- When will I know that they are working?

- How long do I have to take them for?

- Will the depression come back when I stop taking antidepressants?

- How do they interact with other medications?

- What happens if I skip a dose?

- Will I need other therapies in addition to antidepressants?

- Should I be embarrassed?

- Should I let other people know?

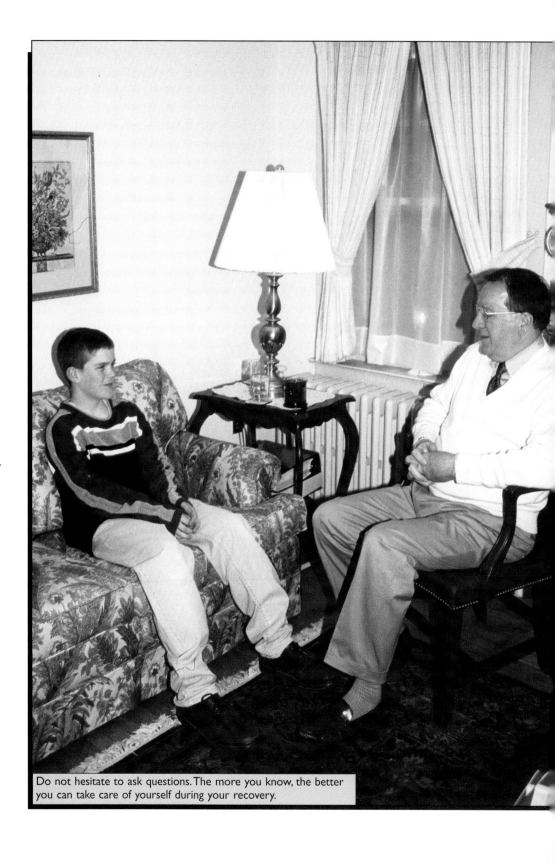

Do not hesitate to ask questions. The more you know, the better you can take care of yourself during your recovery.

Are they addictive?

All of the standard antidepressants that are approved for the treatment of depression are not addictive. An addictive drug makes the person taking it desire increased amounts of that drug. An addictive drug will also make the person feel that he or she needs to keep taking it—as if the person couldn't stop. Studies of patients who have stopped taking antidepressants have shown that the patients do not feel the need to take the antidepressants again. The studies also indicate that while being treated with antidepressants, patients do not desire increased amounts of the drugs.

Will they make me high?

A common physical state of depression is exhaustion. Many people suffering from depression feel zapped of energy. It is not uncommon for patients to start to feel energized or peppy during the early parts of treatment. The restored energy, however, is not to be confused with being high. If you feel dazed or dizzy, you should talk to your psychiatrist or doctor immediately because you may be experiencing an unusual reaction to your medication.

Will they change who I am?

Antidepressants cannot change who you are. They cannot change your life circumstances or the personal characteristics that make you unique. Antidepressants work to change the depressed mood that you are in. Antidepressants help you to feel capable of dealing with issues without feeling overwhelmed. If you feel as if you are reacting to things in a way that would make your "pre-depressed self" uncomfortable, you should discuss it with your psychiatrist or doctor.

How are they given?

Antidepressants can be prescribed alone or in combination with other drugs to increase their effectiveness. It is difficult to know which medication will be most effective in an individual case, so your psychiatrist or doctor may need to take you off one drug and put you on a different one in order to find the prescription that works best for you.

The dosage of the antidepressant varies for each person and for each drug. Doctors work to prescribe the exact dose of an antidepressant so that you can benefit from the drug without suffering too many side effects. The antidepressant dosage usually starts out low and is increased over time until your symptoms of depression have decreased to the desired level. If you take too much of an antidepressant, you could get unnecessary side effects or experience a bad reaction. That is why it's important to follow the instructions that come along with the prescription, which has been formulated with you in mind.

When will I know that they are working?

You probably won't feel immediate results from the antidepressant medication. You should, however, start to feel minor improvement in about one to two weeks. Minor improvement might mean that you are sleeping, eating, or concentrating better than before. You might have more energy or generally feel better. After a few weeks, feelings of hopelessness should fade and you should be better able to deal with problems.

Sometimes the changes are so gradual that you won't be able to notice them yourself, but other people might. Your loved ones might say that you look better or healthier than before. The full benefits of the antidepressants should be felt around four to six weeks after starting medication.

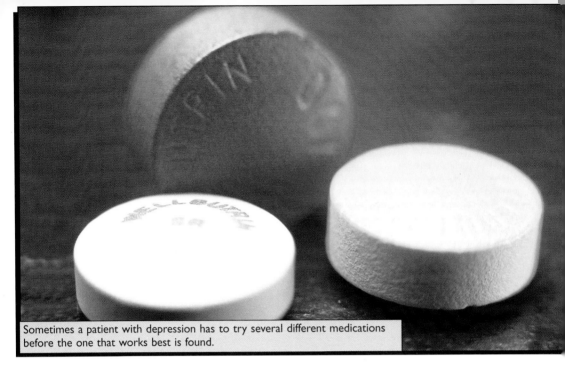

Sometimes a patient with depression has to try several different medications before the one that works best is found.

If there aren't any changes in the depression symptoms after five to seven weeks, a different antidepressant might be prescribed. Since there are several types of antidepressants, there is a good chance that one will work where another has failed. Some patients with depression try several different medications before they find the one that works best for them. Having to wait weeks or months for the medication to work can be very frustrating, but the relief from depression is well worth the wait.

How long do I have to take them for?

The length of time that a patient has to take an antidepressant depends on the individual. Typically, people take antidepressants for eight months or longer. The treatment is usually extended for a few months after the point when they start to feel better. For people suffering from certain kinds of depression, medication may have to be taken indefinitely.

Many patients feel the urge to stop taking the medication after they begin to feel better, or if they think that the medication isn't working. It's important to keep taking the medication because if you stop too early, your original symptoms can return. Some antidepressants can cause bad withdrawal reactions if you stop taking them abruptly. For this reason, your psychiatrist or doctor may decrease the dosage as it is nearing the time to stop taking the drug. Lowering the dosage slowly allows your body the time it needs to adjust in order to avoid a flulike withdrawal.

Will the depression come back when I stop taking antidepressants?

In many cases, with the use of antidepressants, depression can be treated successfully. There is, however, a small chance that depression can return once medication is stopped. If a patient takes antidepressants as suggested by their psychiatrist or doctor, the chance of depression recurring is minimized. If depression reoccurs, it is important to seek treatment as soon as you realize that it has come back.

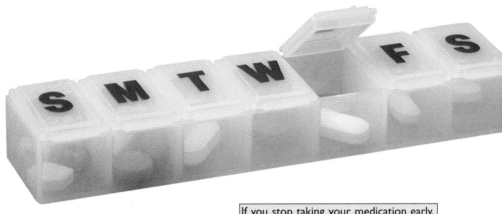

If you stop taking your medication early, your original symptoms can return.

How do they interact with other medications?

All of your health care providers who can prescribe medication should know that you are taking antidepressants. Many drugs that are safe alone can be deadly or cause dangerous side effects when mixed with certain antidepressants. When taken at the same time, some drugs can reduce the effectiveness of your antidepressant. Always get permission from your psychiatrist or doctor before taking any other medication.

What happens if I skip a dose?

If you miss taking your pill, or accidentally take an extra one, you may be changing the level of medication in your system. If the level is too high or too low, it can cause the medication to be less effective. Frequently skipping your medication can make your recovery take longer. You should ask your psychiatrist or doctor what you should do in the event that you accidentally miss a dose.

There are a number of things that can help you remember to take your pills. You can set an alarm clock each day to go off at the time when you should take your pills. Pillboxes with compartments for days of the week are helpful as well. You can buy inexpensive pillboxes at a drugstore or grocery store. At the beginning of the week you can put your pills for each day in each compartment. As you go through the week, you take the pills from the compartment of each day. You can also use a calendar to remind you to take your pills. Try putting a big mark through each day after you have taken your daily dose. Sometimes it works best to use a combination of these techniques in order to help you to remember.

Will I need other therapies in addition to antidepressants?

Many patients receive psychotherapy along with antidepressants. Psychotherapy allows you to discuss personal issues with your psychologist or psychiatrist. While your antidepressant is working to relieve your depressive symptoms, psychotherapy gives you a chance to examine how you feel about everything. It allows you to explore and resolve any concerns or troubles. Psychotherapy has been proven to improve the self-esteem, coping skills, and personal relationships of the patients who participate in it.

Should I be embarrassed?

You should never feel embarrassed because you are depressed. Depression is an illness, and illness is a part of life. People do not get depressed because they are weak or bad. Some of us will never know how painful depression can really be, while others might suffer from diseases far worse than depression. If for some reason, someone makes you feel bad about your illness, tell a parent, teacher, counselor, or your doctor. The person who makes fun of someone who is suffering or ill is really the weak one.

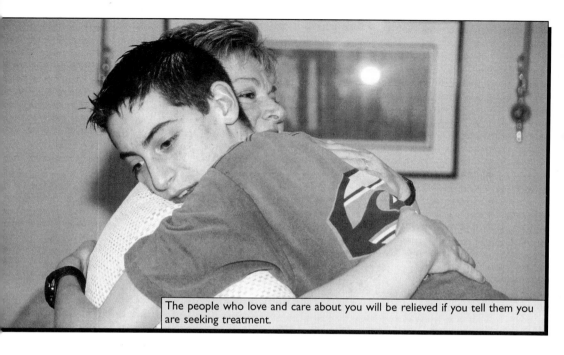

The people who love and care about you will be relieved if you tell them you are seeking treatment.

Should I let other people know?

The people who love and care about you are already aware that you are suffering. They will be relieved to know that you are getting treatment. The people around you who love you and want you to get better are your support system. Their help and concern can make a big difference in your recovery. Sometimes people don't understand how difficult living with depression can be.

Some misinformed people don't think of depression as an illness, but as a state of mind. If you have people within your support system who feel this way, you might have to educate them about depression. It is an added pressure for you to think about, but these people will benefit from your teaching. Your psychiatrist or doctor should be able to supply you with materials or free pamphlets that you can give to your friends or members of your family who might need enlightenment on depression.

Your illness is your business. You don't have to share what you are going through with anyone you don't feel comfortable with. You should never feel as if you have to make excuses for an illness. Speaking with your psychiatrist or doctor about how to deal with your illness in social settings can help you be prepared for anything that might happen. Again, illness is a part of life, and in many cases, so is recovery—you have a lot to look forward to.

4

Side Effects of Antidepressants

All medications can produce side effects. Side effects are what the medication might do to your body in addition to what it is expected to do. When a description sheet of side effects is provided for a medication, it is important to understand that not all people will develop those side effects. The description sheet specifies possible side effects that other people have experienced while using that medication. Many factors can influence the amount of side effects that a person will develop. A person's age, gender, general health, body size, diet, and personal habits can influence the development of side effects while taking a medication. In many cases, the benefits from a medication far outweigh the side effects that are experienced.

Like any medication, antidepressants can produce unwanted side effects. Antidepressant side effects range from merely annoying to very serious. Each patient will experience his or her own reaction to the antidepressant and his or her own range of side effects.

"My doctor believed that my depression was brought about by my grandmother's death. The fact that I didn't want to talk about it made matters worse. When she died, I felt as if a part of me had died, too. I was saving all of my baby-sitting money for the trip that the two of us were going to take during the summer. My family gave me time to grieve, but I didn't come out of the depression.

"My doctor made the decision that I should take medication for my depression. He said that the medication might help to relieve the sadness so that I could talk about it without being overcome by grief. My mother and I sat in his office while he explained the use of antidepressants.

"After the talk, my doctor handed us a sheet that listed the side effects of the antidepressant I would be taking. I gasped as I read the long list. I couldn't believe it . . . was I really going

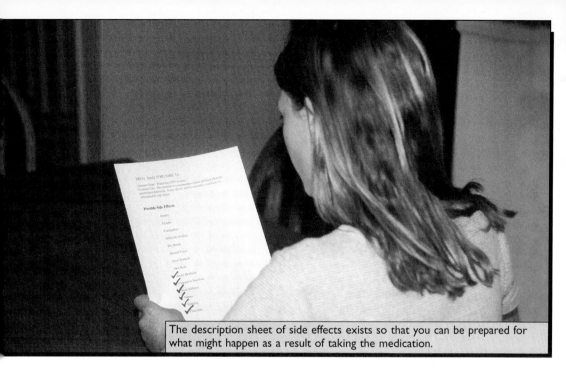

The description sheet of side effects exists so that you can be prepared for what might happen as a result of taking the medication.

to get insomnia? I wasn't sleeping well already. The nervousness and nausea ... would I experience that, too? The point was that I wasn't feeling good to begin with. I was tired and suffered from nausea already. The list scared me. Why take the medication if it could cause the very things that I was already suffering with?"
—Emily, sixteen

The description sheet of an antidepressant's possible side effects is not meant to scare you. It exists so that you can be prepared for what might happen as a result of taking the medication. If you know what might happen, you can be prepared in case it does, rather than being confused as to what is happening. When reading your description sheet about the possible side effects, familiarize yourself with what may happen. Remember, though, that while some people may experience the side effects, others will not. In addition, some people may experience just one or two side effects, whereas others experience five or six. Most side effects of antidepressants are manageable and will disappear over time or after the medication is stopped.

It is a good idea to sit down with your doctor and review the possible side effects sheet together. Ask your doctor to put a check beside any side effects that you must call in to report about, should you experience them. Your psychiatrist or doctor will take an active interest in how you are responding to the medication.

During your treatment, your doctor may frequently ask you about side effects. You should mention any changes or new sensations that you are feeling. If the side effects aren't normal, your doctor will make medication adjustments so that the changes or new sensations don't get worse. Any unusual side effects, ones that interfere with your general health and well-being, should be reported to your psychiatrist or doctor immediately so that your dosage can be adjusted.

Side Effects Specific to the Antidepressant Groups

Research on the four main groups of anti-depressants has shown that there are some side effects that are commonly reported in each specific group. This means that people taking different drugs from the TCA group are reporting common side effects, and people taking MAOIs or SSRIs are, too.

Possible side effects of MAOIs

Research has found that if you take certain medications, food, and beverages while being treated with any of the MAOIs, you could raise your blood pressure to a dangerously high level. Your psychiatrist or doctor will give you an extensive list of medications, foods, and beverages to avoid during your treatment. Everyone taking MAOIs must accept restrictions in order to avoid the potentially dangerous side effect of severe high blood pressure. Signs of a bad reaction include increased blood pressure levels, headache, nausea, vomiting, and seizures. This kind of reaction requires immediate medical attention. You can avoid these side effects by avoiding the medications, foods, and beverages on the list provided by your psychiatrist or doctor.

A common side effect of stopping MAOI treatment abruptly is the onset of withdrawal symptoms. These symptoms are flulike and include nausea and vomiting. You can avoid withdrawal symptoms by following your psychiatrist's or doctor's plan for lowering your medication dosage rather than stopping abruptly.

Possible side effects of TCAs

Side effects common to the TCA group include dry mouth, dizziness when changing positions, and drowsiness. To avoid dry mouth, it's good to drink a lot of water. To avoid dizziness when changing positions, it works to move slowly. Your psychiatrist or doctor might suggest taking the TCA at night if it is causing you to feel drowsy. This will help you to sleep at night and allow you to be more alert during the day. TCAs can also mix badly with certain medications and beverages. Your psychiatrist or doctor will provide you with a list of medications and beverages to avoid taking while on TCAs.

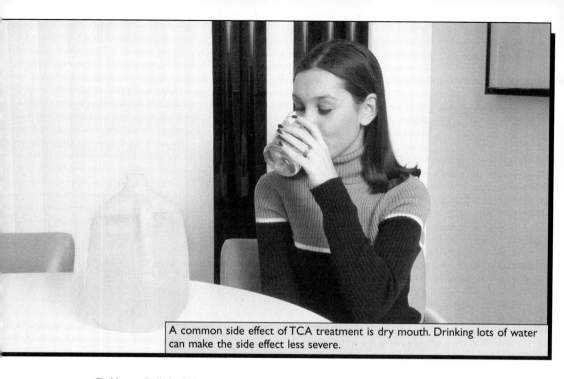

A common side effect of TCA treatment is dry mouth. Drinking lots of water can make the side effect less severe.

Like MAOIs, stopping your treatment abruptly with TCAs can cause withdrawal symptoms. Symptoms of TCA withdrawal can include nausea, headache, nightmares, and feeling ill. To avoid withdrawal symptoms, follow your psychiatrist's or doctor's treatment plan.

Possible side effects of SSRIs

SSRIs tend to have fewer side effects than MAOIs and TCAs. Side effects common to the SSRIs include headache, insomnia, and nervousness. The headaches will eventually subside or disappear with time. You can speak with your psychiatrist or doctor about the best time to take your pill if you are suffering from insomnia. If you develop nervousness that doesn't subside over time, your psychiatrist or doctor will adjust your dosage to relieve the side effect. You should also ask to be given a list of medications to avoid while taking SSRIs.

As with MAOIs and TCAs, withdrawal symptoms from ending treatment abruptly can also occur with SSRIs. It is important to follow your psychiatrist's or doctor's treatment plan to avoid possible symptoms.

Possible side effects of the other antidepressants

The side effects commonly reported for this group are a combination of the effects found in the three named groups. These effects include dry mouth, dizziness, headaches, nervousness, or insomnia. As with the three named groups, side effects can be avoided or managed by following instructions on how to deal with those side effects. Your psychiatrist or doctor will give you important information regarding the specific drug that has been prescribed to you from this group.

5

Making Depression Easier

Living with depression on a day-to-day basis can be very difficult. There are some activities, though, that can help you to relieve some of the difficulty. If you are receiving psychotherapy as well as medication, you should ask your psychiatrist or psychologist for the activities that he or she might recommend first.

Practice Patience

All throughout your treatment it is best that you allow yourself patience. Sometimes things work, and sometimes no matter how hard you try, they don't work. It might help to repeat a saying to yourself that helps you to hang on; repeating and believing something such as "Hang in there, it will get better" will serve as effective self-support.

Try to Recognize Negative Thinking

Depression makes you think negative thoughts. It is a good practice to pay attention to the kind of thoughts that your mind creates. When the thoughts are negative, remind yourself that those thoughts are part of the depression—that they are not rational, and at some point during treatment they will go away. When you find that you have a positive thought, give yourself credit. The positive thoughts will hopefully replace the negative thoughts as you respond to treatment. If at any time your negative thoughts lead you to consider suicide, tell your parents and doctor immediately.

Activities for the Mind

The following suggestions have been used by patients to relieve the day-to-day difficulties of depression. If some activities don't work for you, keep trying until you find ones that do work for you.

Write

Keep a journal of your day-to-day experiences. What you will remember about a

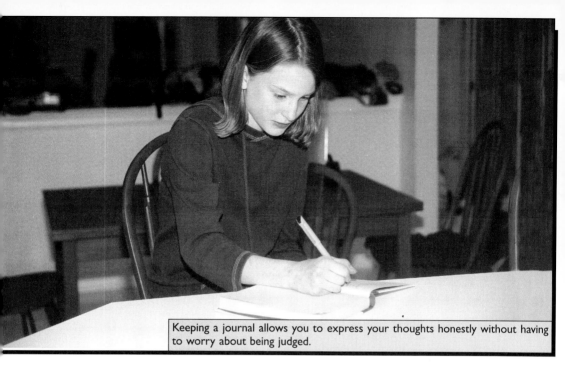

Keeping a journal allows you to express your thoughts honestly without having to worry about being judged.

particular experience can be totally different from how you felt on the day that it was happening. A journal allows you to put your feelings down on paper where you will not forget them. Keeping a journal allows you the chance to be totally honest without the fear of someone judging your feelings. You are also in control of the thoughts that you put down and how you want to express them. In the process of writing about your feelings, you allow yourself to move on to other things because you have examined how you felt and then put it down on paper. You can always refer to the tough days that you wrote about in your journal to see the progress that you have made since then.

Read

Reading is a wonderful activity for the mind. Reading other people's thoughts can keep your mind from dwelling on your depression. Read anything and everything that interests you. You can even read biographies about people who have had depression, which can allow you to see how they coped with the difficulties. There is a wonderful world of books waiting for you to explore, and if you start reading now you will discover what a life-long, healthy habit reading can be.

Talk

If you find that something makes you nervous or anxious, talk to someone about it. It helps if the person is a good listener, but sometimes the simple act of saying something out loud can make all the difference between feeling anxious or feeling relieved. If there are problems or issues that you have trouble facing, go to a friend or loved one and ask for support.

Set the right kind of goals

Goals give people something to work toward. Setting goals can be extremely difficult while suffering from depression. The various depressive moods can keep a person from caring about the future. Choosing goals that are difficult to obtain can put too much pressure on you. Set simple goals, and go easy on yourself if depression keeps you from accomplishing them.

List your goals

Making a list of things to do each day is a good exercise. On some days, your depression may be so severe that you won't want to get out of bed. On a day like that, your to-do list could be as simple as "Get out of bed. Take a shower." At the end of the day, when you have done those two things, you should feel good knowing that you accomplished the goals on your list. Don't get discouraged if you don't get to all of the goals on your daily lists. Goals that you didn't get to one day can be put on another list when the time is right. You can also write your to-do list in your journal; that way you can see all of the things that you have accomplished and the things that you have yet to do.

Make a feel-good tape or CD

There are songs that can make us feel better even in the most desperate of moments. That is the gift that music gives to us. We all have different favorites, but they all work the same way. You hear that song, and you feel touched—you might even feel hopeful. At the very least, you no longer feel alone. The process of making a feel-good tape or CD can be as fun as listening to it, so make as many as you want. When you feel the need to be lifted, play the tape or CD, and allow yourself to enjoy it. If there are lyrics to the music, sing along with them. The act of singing allows the mind and the body to connect, which is very healthy. Don't worry about your singing skills, just breathe and belt it out.

Activities for the Whole Self

Participate in feel-good activities

Mild exercise, going to the movies, playing an instrument, or participating in a sport are wonderful activities for the body and brain. Activities that make you feel good can be anything from reorganizing your closet to jogging around the block. Try to stay away from any activities that might make you think negative thoughts about yourself.

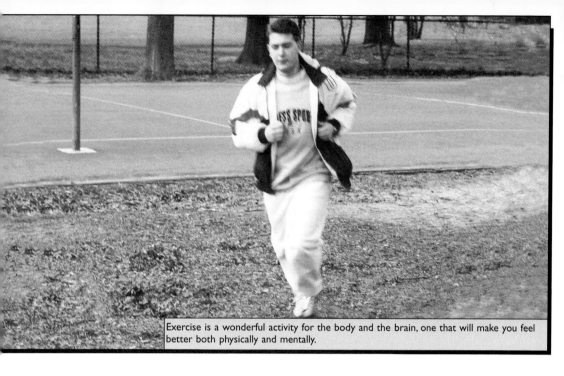

Exercise is a wonderful activity for the body and the brain, one that will make you feel better both physically and mentally.

Be around people who make you feel better

It's easy to want to isolate yourself during depression. Sometimes you might feel guilty for not being happy, but you have to remind yourself that guilt is one of the negative feelings that might come along with depression. You need to find positive thoughts to replace the guilt. Being around people who are positive can be very uplifting for the mood. If you find that a particular family member makes you feel good to be around, visit with them. You don't have to talk if you don't want to—you can ask if it's okay for you to sit and listen. Hearing the voice and the words of a positive person can be very uplifting. If it feels good to confide in that person, share your thoughts with him or her. You can even ask for a hug.

Practice meditating

Meditation allows a person to focus his or her thoughts while feeling relaxed. There are several different ways to meditate. There are a variety of books that can help you to find which meditation method is the best for you. You might find that sometimes it is harder or easier to practice meditation depending on your depressive state, but as you respond to treatment, meditation should get easier.

Help for Your Family and Friends

The effects of depression are felt not only by the depressed person but by his or her family and friends as well. Although people suffering from depression don't mean to, they can often frustrate their loved ones and put distance between themselves and family or friends. Family members and friends must try not to take it personally. They might be justified in feeling mad sometimes, but they must get over it. They should remind themselves that their loved one is suffering from a very real and serious illness.

Family and friends must also release themselves from feeling responsible for making the depressed person feel better. Love, caring, and laughter are wonderful for the spirit, but someone who is depressed will also need psychological and medical attention to get over his or her depression. Here is a list of requests that you can use to help your family and friends understand what you may be going through.

■ Please do not accuse me of faking an illness. I want to get better and I need your support. I can't just snap out of this. I need your understanding, patience, and affection.

■ Sometimes I need to hear that you believe I will get better—that I need to be patient while being treated because it will all get better.

■ If I tell you how I feel, please do not tell me that my feelings aren't right, but instead offer me hope.

■ If I should mention suicide, if I question the point of being alive, please tell my parents or my therapist.

■ Even though I often say no, please

invite me for walks, outings, the movies, and things that you like to do. If I finally say yes, please don't make a big deal out of it. Let me accompany you without too many pressures.

▬ Please do not let the fact that I have depression make you depressed. It's okay for you to enjoy life and have fun even while I am depressed.

▬ Please encourage me to do the healthy activities that I used to like doing, but if I can't do them, tell me that it's okay.

▬ It would be nice if you could learn more about my condition. My psychiatrist (doctor or psychologist) has given me a pamphlet that you can read, which will help you to understand what I am going through.

"This may sound weird, but I think that my depression made me a better person. It took three years to be treated and get rid of my depression. During those three years, I experienced many successes and failures, but those experiences taught me how to deal with life's issues.

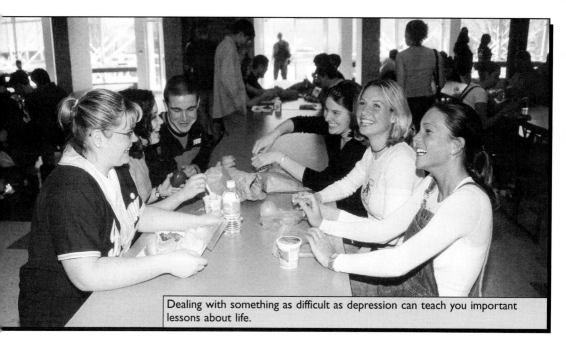

Dealing with something as difficult as depression can teach you important lessons about life.

"I learned how to take better care of myself. Every time I took a moment to take care of my needs, I felt better. It is important that you don't let depression overshadow the simple things that your body needs in order to function properly. I realize the importance of eating healthy, energizing foods and getting enough sleep. Both of these things—a good diet and the right amount of rest—can help you to work toward having a clear, unburdened mind. The little things, such as taking walks in the yard or playing my guitar, made me feel special, too. I still use my pill alarm, but when I used to take my medication, I now take vitamins. It helps remind me of what I have been through and how I am working toward staying healthy.

"I am much better at coping with issues now than I was before the depression. The moment that I notice I am having difficulties with something, I talk about it with someone who cares. I also keep writing in my journal. Keeping a journal allows me to face things with a clearer head. Before I started using a journal, my random thoughts just added to the dark clouds in my mind. Now, by writing about my problems or issues, I can organize my thoughts. I also read a lot more books than before. I get excited thinking about all of the books at the bookstore and the library. If I am ever curious about something, there is most likely a book written about it.

"Having gone through depression, I am more sensitive toward other people and the problems that they might be experiencing. I know that even though someone might seem all right, it might not be true. Someone can be smiling on the outside, but feel totally isolated and miserable on the inside. Depression helped me to understand that there are some illnesses that you can't see just by looking at someone.

"I may have learned the most important lesson of all because of my depression, and that is to never give up. No matter what, we all face difficulties, so it's important to think of each difficulty as a learning experience. Each experience

can offer you lessons about life. By learning from those lessons, you can become a better person."
—*Jackie, seventeen*

By taking an active interest in your recovery, you will find depression a little easier to deal with. Once your family and friends understand what you are going through, you won't feel as alone and isolated as many people suffering from depression do. Maintain the medication instructions that your psychiatrist or doctor has given you, and try to be honest and open with your feelings—no matter what. Even though it seems like a lot of work, hopefully you will be rewarded by your struggles, and one day you will wake up without the dark clouds in your mind.

Glossary

amphetamine   A class of drugs used to stimulate the nervous system.

antidepressant   A class of drugs used to treat depressive mental disorders.

depression   A condition of general emotional unhappiness and withdrawal.

depressive disorder   A disturbance in the brain resulting in ranges of depression.

insomnia   The inability to sleep, or chronic sleeplessness.

lithium   A drug of the antimanic class that is sometimes used to treat certain depressions.

MAOIs (Monoamine Oxidase Inhibitors)   The earliest group of drugs to be used in the treatment of depression.

meditation   A method of relaxation that involves deep breathing and focused thoughts.

mental disorder   A disturbance in the brain.

psychiatrist A physician who practices psychiatry. Psychiatrists can prescribe medication.

psychiatry The practice and science of treating mental diseases.

psychologist A specialist in psychology.

psychology The science of the mind, mental states, and processes.

psychotherapy The science of using psychological techniques to cure psychological disorders.

side effect An additional effect of a medication that has nothing to do with the purpose for which it is being prescribed.

SSRIs (Selective Serotonin Reuptake Inhibitors) The third oldest group of antidepressants, known to have fewer side effects than MAOIs and TCAs. Referred to as new antidepressants.

support system A group of people working together to provide support.

TCAs (Tricyclic Antidepressants) The second oldest antidepressant group. Known to have fewer side effects than MAOIs.

therapy The treatment of a disease.

withdrawal Physical and psychological symptoms that can occur when medication is stopped.

Where to Go for Help

In the United States

American Academy of Child and Adolescent Psychiatry
3615 Wisconsin Avenue NW
Washington, DC 20016-3007
(800) 333-7636
Web site: http://www.aacap.org

American Psychiatric Association
1400 K Street NW
Washington, DC 20005
(202) 682-6000
Web site: http://www.psych.org

American Psychological Association
750 First Street NE
Washington, DC 20002-4242
(202) 336-5500
Web site: http://www.apa.org

Center for Mental Health Services (CMHS)
P.O. Box 42490
Washington, DC 20015
(800) 789-CMHS (2647)
Web site: http://www.mentalhealth.org

National Alliance for the Mentally Ill (NAMI)
2107 Wilson Boulevard, Suite 300
Arlington, VA 22201-3042
(800) 950-NAMI (6264)
Web site: http://www.nami.org

National Mental Health Association (NMHA)
1021 Prince Street
Alexandria, VA 22314-2971
(800) 969-NMHA
Web site: http://www.nmha.org

In Canada

Canadian Mental Health Association
2160 Yonge Street, 3rd Floor
Toronto, ON M4S 2Z3
(416) 484-7750

Canadian Psychiatric Association
260-441 MacLaren Street
Ottawa, ON K2P 2H3
(613) 234-2815
Web site: http://cpa.medical.org

Web Sites

American Foundation for Suicide Prevention (AFSP)
http://www.afsp.org

Internet Mental Health
http://www.mentalhealth.com

Suicide Awareness, Voices of Education (SAVE)
http://www.save.org

For Further Reading

Cobain, Bev, and Jeff Tolbert (Illustrator). *When Nothing Matters Anymore: A Survival Guide for Depressed Teens.* Minneapolis, MN: Free Spirit Press, 1998.

Garland, E. Jane. *Depression Is the Pits, but I'm Getting Better: A Guide for Adolescents.* New York: Magination Press, 1998.

Jaffe, Steven L., and B. Joan McClure. *Prozac and Other Antidepressants.* Broomall, PA: Chelsea House Publishers, 1999.

Klebanoff, Susan, Ellen Luborsky, and Andy Cooke (Illustrator). *Ups and Downs: How to Beat the Blues and Teen Depression* (Plugged In). Los Angeles, CA: Price Stern Sloan Publishing, 1999.

Simpson, Carolyn, and Penelope Hall. *RX: Reading and Following the Directions for All Kinds of Medications.* New York: Rosen Publishing Group, 1994.

Index

About the Author
Holly Cefrey attended the University of Nebraska before moving to New York. She is a freelance writer, researcher, and artist.

Photo Credits
Cover by Brian Silak; pp. 2, 8, 17, 23, 26, 35, 39, 47, 55 by Maura Boruchow; p. 13 by Brian Silak; pp. 21, 30 by Custom Medical Stock Photo; p. 32 © Corbis; p. 43 by Debra Rothenberg; p. 51 by Ira Fox.

Series Design
Geri Giordano

Layout
Danielle Goldblatt